PUBERTY EDUCATION FOR YOUR CHILDREN

A Compassionate Guide to Puberty Education for Your Growing Stars

JAY C. WATSON

TABLE OF CONTENT

INTRODUCTION

Understanding the Importance of Puberty Education

Embarking on the journey of puberty with your children is an important milestone in the tapestry of motherhood. Understanding the significance of puberty education is not only about imparting knowledge; it is a critical act of empowerment. Puberty symbolizes a transitional stage in a child's life, comprising physical, emotional, and social changes. Armed with information, both parents and children can traverse this complicated environment with confidence and grace.

Empowering Through Knowledge:
Puberty education builds the basis for empowerment. It prepares youngsters with an awareness of the changes their bodies will endure, encouraging a feeling of control and ownership over their experiences. Knowledge becomes a strong tool, helping people to make educated choices, accept their growing identities,

and continue on the road of self-discovery with resilience.

Building a Foundation of Trust:
The foundation of puberty education is based on trust. As parents, your job goes beyond that of educators; you are mentors and confidants. By discussing facts freely and honestly, you establish a trusting connection with your children. This trust becomes a critical pillar, enabling children to seek help and communicate their worries as they negotiate the difficulties and wonders of adolescence.

Creating a Safe and Open Environment for Discussions

Creating a safe and open space for talks is the cornerstone of good puberty education. The house becomes a refuge where inquiries are accepted and curiosity is cherished. Fostering an environment of open communication allows children to voice their views, worries, and anxieties without fear of judgment. It converts the learning process into a shared adventure, increasing the parent-child link.

Bridging the Generation Gap:
Puberty generally presents a subtle change in the interactions between parents and children. Creating an open atmosphere helps bridge the age divide, allowing for meaningful talks that transcend the roles of authority and adolescence. It prepares the way for understanding, empathy, and shared experiences, building a relationship that withstands the hardships of this transitional age.

Embracing Diversity of Experience:
Every child's experience of puberty is unique. Creating an open atmosphere entails acknowledging and respecting the variety of these experiences. Acknowledge that each kid may have different questions, concerns, and deadlines. By accepting this uniqueness, you promote the concept that there is no one-size-fits-all approach to puberty and that every experience is legitimate.

Setting the Stage for an Empowered Puberty JourneyAs we continue on this examination of puberty education for your children, let the awareness of its significance be a compass leading you through the subtleties of growing. Creating a secure and open atmosphere is the key that opens doors to meaningful talks, shared discoveries, and a pleasant transition into this transformational era. May this introduction create the basis for a journey filled with insight, connection, and the pleasure of learning together.

Breaking the Stigma:
In our investigation of puberty education, it is crucial to tear down the walls of stigma that may surround this normal era of life. Open talks about puberty help to normalize the issue, providing an atmosphere where youngsters feel comfortable approaching their parents with questions or concerns. By removing cultural taboos, parents become allies in helping their children accept their developing bodies with confidence.

Celebrating development and change:

Puberty is a celebration of development and change. By establishing an open place for talks, parents have the chance to celebrate these developments with their children. Encourage children to enjoy the beauty of their changing selves and establish a positive outlook on the trip ahead. This celebration extends beyond the physical changes; it incorporates the growth of character, resilience, and a greater awareness of self.

Setting Expectations for the Parental Role Guides Through the Unknown:

As parents, consider yourself mentors through the unexplored realms of adolescence. Your responsibility is not to have all the answers but to give constant support, understanding, and direction. Puberty education is a joint endeavor when both parents and children go on a path of learning together. Embrace the role of navigator, helping your children navigate the oceans of change with knowledge and compassion.

Fostering a lifetime discourse:

Puberty education signals the beginning of a lifetime discourse between parents and children. By establishing expectations for continued talks, you develop a foundation for open communication that endures into adolescence and beyond. This discourse provides a crucial avenue for addressing new issues, exchanging experiences, and fostering a relationship founded on trust and mutual understanding.

The Puberty Adventure Map:

Think of puberty as an adventure with an expanding map. As parents, you hold the map, leading your children through the twists and turns of this voyage. The map isn't simply a series of directions; it's a collective effort, marked by shared experiences, fun, and the odd difficulty. Embrace the journey ahead with a feeling of interest, knowing that each step offers new discoveries and potential for progress.

In conclusion, this investigation of puberty education is more than a guide; it is a promise of empowerment. Through understanding and open conversation, parents enable their children to embrace puberty not as a terrifying time but as a transformational and fulfilling experience. The trip ahead is a joint one, full of learning, love, and the pleasure of growing together.

As we set sail into the heart of puberty education, let the breezes of understanding and openness fill our sails. May our journey be defined by shared insights, celebrations of development, and the delight of discovery. Together, parents and children navigate the waves of puberty, building a relationship that withstands the tides of change. Embrace the adventure—it's a tour of love, progress, and the beauty of shared understanding.

Chapter 1
WHAT IS PUBERTY?

Defining Puberty

Puberty, like the first light of morning, symbolizes the beginning of a transforming journey. It is a natural and universal process by which a kid matures into a teenager and finally into adulthood. Puberty comprises a sequence of physiological, emotional, and psychological changes that prepare a person for the challenges of adult life. In essence, it is the awakening of the body, mind, and soul to the glories of adulthood.

Biological Alchemy:

At its foundation, puberty is a biological alchemy controlled by hormones. The endocrine system, comparable to an internal symphony conductor, produces hormones that initiate a cascade of changes. These changes materialize physically, emotionally, and socially, laying the foundation for the individual's path towards self-discovery and maturity.

<u>**Physical and emotional changes**</u>
The Canvas of Physical Transformation:
Picture the body as a canvas, and puberty as the brushstroke that alters it. Physically, puberty presents a multitude of changes that are unique to each person. In boys, there's the growth spurt, the deepening of the voice, and the appearance of facial hair—a witness to the passage from boyhood to manhood. Girls undergo the growth of breasts, the commencement of menstruation, and a gradual rise in height—a delicate progression from girlhood to womanhood.

The Emotional Symphony of Adolescence: Puberty isn't merely a physical change; it's also an emotional symphony. Emotions, much like musical notes, grow deeper, more subtle, and sometimes unexpected. Adolescents may find themselves on a rollercoaster of feelings—joy, perplexity, excitement, and contemplation. Understanding and navigating this emotional terrain is a critical component of the puberty journey, both for teenagers and the guiding hands of their parents.

Hormonal Choreography:
Imagine hormones as the choreographers of this big dance called puberty. The pituitary gland, the director of ceremonies, orchestrates the release of hormones like estrogen and testosterone. These hormones drive the development of secondary sexual traits, changing the individual's physical appearance and laying the path for the transition into adulthood.

Growth as a Tapestry:
Growth throughout puberty is like constructing a tapestry. Each thread symbolizes a distinct component of development—height, body composition, and the fine nuances of reproductive maturity. The tapestry expands not just in physical dimensions but also in the depth of experiences, relationships, and self-awareness. Puberty becomes a period of discovery, analogous to an artist producing a masterpiece on the canvas of one's own life.

As we dig into the core of puberty, consider it a dance—a dance of biological rhythms, emotional melodies, and physical modifications. The definitions are not static; they are verses in a poetic story, each unique to the person. Puberty is not simply a period of life; it's a vivid, dynamic journey—an unfolding epic where each individual becomes both the narrator and the protagonist. May this inquiry inspire parents and children to accept the rhythms of puberty with curiosity, understanding, and the pleasure of growing.

Chapter 2
WHEN DOES PUBERTY START?

Signs of Puberty

The advent of puberty heralds a foreshadowing of change—a whisper in the wind heralding the beginning of a remarkable journey. Signs of puberty commonly occur between the ages of 8 and 13, changing from person to person. One of the early heralds is the growth spurt, a subtle lengthening of limbs that lays the foundation for the physical alterations to come.

Emergence of secondary sexual characteristics: puberty unfurls its canvas via the emergence of secondary sexual characteristics. In males, this may involve the deepening of the voice, the growth of facial hair, and the expansion of the Adam's apple. For females, the growth of breasts, the advent of menstruation, and changes in body form become the brushstrokes that create the image of adolescence. These signals represent the delicate dance of hormones, directing the change from infancy to maturity.

Variations in Puberty Onset

Puberty, much like a celestial event, follows its own distinct timeframes for each person. While some may feel the first whispers of change early, others may begin on this road a little later. Variations in puberty onset are determined by a mix of genetic, environmental, and individual variables.

Early bloomers vs. late bloomers:

Imagine a garden where flowers bloom at various times. Early bloomers, experiencing puberty ahead of their contemporaries, may negotiate the panorama of change with a feeling of individuality. On the other hand, late bloomers take a different route, experiencing the marvels of puberty at their own leisure. Both early and late bloomers add to the various beauty of the garden, indicating that there is no one or 'correct' timing for the start of puberty.

Puberty as an unexpected symphony:

Picture puberty as an unexpected symphony, where each instrument plays its notes in a distinct rhythm. The variations in onset form part of this symphony, providing a rich and complex composition. Embracing these distinctions is not just a celebration of uniqueness but also an understanding that the path into puberty is as distinctive as a fingerprint.

Parental Support Through variances:

For parents, helping children through the variances in puberty onset includes a delicate dance of understanding and comfort. Being aware of your child's emotional environment, giving a listening ear, and providing age-appropriate knowledge will help them manage the uncertainty. The beauty comes in the unpredictability—each note, each shift, adds to the harmonic harmony of growing up.

As we study when puberty begins, let's consider it a cosmic dance, a choreography of development and change that unfolds individually for each person. Signs of puberty become the constellations in the night sky, tracing the journey into adolescence. Embracing variances in onset becomes an invitation to dance to the unexpected symphony of growing up, honoring the richness that variety provides to the ever-evolving fabric of existence.

Chapter 3
BODY CHANGES

<u>**Changes in Boys**</u>

1. **The Metamorphosis of Boyhood**: As boys start on the journey of puberty, their bodies undergo a spectacular metamorphosis—a move from the familiar terrain of boyhood to the undiscovered areas of adolescence. One of the key indications of puberty in males is the growth spurt. Like budding branches reaching for the sky, males endure a dramatic rise in height, signaling the start of physical transformation.

2. **The Symphony of Vocal Evolution**: Imagine the voice as an instrument tuning itself to a new tune. In males, the deepening of the voice is a substantial development. The once-high tones of childhood progressively give way to a deeper resonance—an audible witness to the hormonal symphony directing the metamorphosis from boy to young man.

3. The **Emergence of Facial Hair**: Picture facial hair as the brushstrokes that create the canvas of youth. During puberty, males may observe the growth of facial hair, marking the advent of a more adult physical look. This alteration, frequently accompanied by a feeling of pride, becomes a visible emblem of the journey into masculinity.

Changes in girls

For girls, the journey of puberty is a blossoming—a delicate unfurling of petals that symbolizes the transition from childhood to adolescence. One of the notable changes is the growth of breasts. As if emerging from a nap, the chest region experiences changes, signifying the start of puberty and the steady growth of the body.

1. Menstruation:
The Rhythmic Cycle of Womanhood

Menstruation, a characteristic of female adolescence, exposes females to the cyclical cycle of womanhood. This deep and natural process shows the preparation of the reproductive system. Understanding menstruation becomes a key component of puberty education, helping girls negotiate this portion of their bodily journey with confidence and awareness.

2. Changes in Body Form: Imagine the body as a sculpture taking form. During puberty, females suffer changes in body composition, including the expansion of hips and a shift in fat distribution. These adjustments lead to a more mature and feminine silhouette—a physical expression of the complicated dance of hormones directing them through puberty.

Parental counsel Through bodily changes: Navigating the bodily changes in boys and girls needs parental counsel that is both knowledgeable and sensitive. Providing age-appropriate information, answering concerns freely, and maintaining a supportive atmosphere are vital. Parents become the steadfast anchors, bringing confidence as their children sail the often tumultuous but awe-inspiring seas of physical development.

The beauty of variety:

As we go into the chapter on physical modifications, let's appreciate the beauty of variety. Puberty is a journey distinguished by distinct timetables and unique alterations. Every change, whether in boys or girls, adds to the colorful tapestry of growing up. Embrace the canvas of puberty as a work of art, where each brushstroke contributes to the beauty of the unfolding masterpiece.

In the investigation of physical changes, may parents and children discover illumination—a guiding light that turns the often enigmatic path of puberty into a shared adventure. The canvas of puberty, filled with changes in boys and girls, becomes a monument to the great variety and tenacity of the human spirit. As we move through this chapter, let the colors of understanding, joy, and empathy brighten the way ahead.

Chapter 4
HORMONES AND THEIR ROLE

Explaining Hormones

The Chemical Messengers:

At the core of the puberty symphony are hormones—a sophisticated ensemble of chemical messengers coordinating the multidimensional shift from infancy to adolescence. These signals, secreted by the endocrine glands, function like conductors, sculpting the physical, emotional, and psychological landscapes of puberty.

Estrogen and Testosterone:

The Principal PlayersPicture estrogen and testosterone as the major musicians in this hormonal symphony. In females, estrogen takes center stage, leading to the development of secondary sexual characteristics, controlling the menstrual cycle, and contributing to the general maturity of the reproductive system. In males, testosterone emerges as the lead, affecting the growth of facial hair, deepening of the voice, and the development of muscles—a monument to the passage from boyhood to manhood.

Emotional Rollercoaster: Hormones and Mood Swings

The Canvas of Emotional Expression:

As hormones swell and ebb like the tides, they produce an emotional canvas where teenagers express the complexities of their changing inner worlds. Mood swings become the brushstrokes on this canvas—a kaleidoscope of emotions ranging from elation and enthusiasm to perplexity and reflection. Understanding the emotional rollercoaster is crucial to managing the delicate dance of hormones throughout puberty.

Navigating the Peaks and Valleys:

Imagine the emotional landscape as a topography of peaks and valleys. Hormones, like fickle winds, may carry teenagers to dizzying heights of ecstasy or hurl them into the depths of doubt. Navigating these emotional peaks and troughs involves not only self-awareness but also the compassionate direction of parents, who become the steadfast lighthouses amid the turbulent seas of adolescence.

Communication as the Compass: Communication becomes the compass that leads teenagers and parents through the emotional rollercoaster of puberty. Open and honest interactions establish a bridge, encouraging understanding and empathy. Parents, with their wealth of experience, become navigators, helping their children sail over the emotional waves with resilience and a sense of self-discovery.

Embracing the Symphony:
In the magnificent symphony of puberty, hormones are the notes that build a song of development and change. Rather than perceiving mood swings as interruptions, imagine them as a dynamic dance—a movement that creates character, resilience, and emotional intelligence. Embracing this hormonal symphony entails recognizing the beauty in the variety of emotions

and accepting that, much like a piece of music, the journey through puberty is richer by its subtle composition.

Parental Support as the Conductor's Baton:
As the hormonal symphony develops, parents step into the position of conductors, carrying the baton of support and understanding. Providing a secure environment for emotional expression, providing comfort during periods of doubt, and enjoying the highs of delight create a harmonic setting where the dance of hormones changes into a beautiful and profound journey of self-discovery.

Harmonizing the Hormonal Melody:
In our investigation of hormones and their function, let's consider it a harmonic melody—an ever-evolving song that characterizes the puberty experience. Understanding hormones becomes not merely a medical lesson but a tool for accessing the emotional depth of puberty. May the dance of hormones and mood swings be addressed with

compassion, discussion, and the harmonizing efforts of parents and teenagers alike.

Building Emotional Intelligence:
Navigating the emotional rollercoaster of puberty gives teenagers a unique chance to build emotional intelligence. Parents, as mentors, may nurture this intelligence by fostering self-reflection and helping their children verbalize and comprehend their emotions. The capacity to detect and control emotions becomes a key life skill that goes into puberty.

Empathy as the Bridge:
Empathy acts as the bridge linking parents and teenagers over the emotional terrain of puberty. By placing themselves in their children's position, parents may better comprehend the struggles and successes of the hormonal journey. This sympathetic connection develops trust, enables open communication, and enhances the parent-child link during a period of great emotional exploration.

Weathering the Storms:
Resilience, like a solid vessel, helps teenagers withstand the storms of emotional highs and lows. Parents play a vital role in cultivating this resilience by highlighting the temporary nature of mood swings, creating a feeling of self-awareness, and reinforcing the concept that obstacles are chances for development. Through this nurturing, teenagers learn the fortitude to sail the unpredictable oceans of emotions.

Encouraging Positive Coping Techniques: Teaching adolescents positive coping techniques helps them handle the emotional turmoil successfully. Whether via artistic outlets, physical activities, or mindfulness practices, these coping techniques become the lifebuoys that help teenagers remain afloat throughout hard emotional times. Parents operate as mentors, supporting their children in developing coping mechanisms that connect with their specific needs.

Understanding the enormous influence of hormones on emotions helps parents approach the emotional rollercoaster with tolerance, understanding, and a deep respect for the difficult journey their children are traversing. By embracing the dance of hormones and mood swings, parents become not simply witnesses but active players in a symphony that eventually determines the resilience, character, and emotional well-being of their teenagers. May this continual harmony be a source of connection, progress, and shared understanding throughout the great journey of puberty.

Chapter 5
MENSTRUATION FOR GIRLS

What is Menstruation?

Menstruation, a wonderful element of the female reproductive system, emerges as a delicate dance—a rhythmic manifestation of nature's perfection. It symbolizes the body's preparedness for prospective pregnancy, arranging a monthly symphony that becomes an important part of a woman's life. Picture menstruation as the smooth rhythm of a timeless tune, a pleasant reminder of the cyclical essence of existence.

Understanding the Menstrual Cycle:

At the center of menstruation is the menstrual cycle, a complex interplay of hormones directing the development of an egg and the preparation of the uterus for possible conception. The cycle comprises several stages, each contributing to the orchestration of this natural and crucial activity. Understanding the menstrual cycle becomes a powerful tool, helping females embrace their reproductive health with knowledge and confidence.

The menstrual cycle is a rhythmic journey that reveals the secrets of a woman's body. It begins with the first day of menstruation, marking Day 1, and continues until the next month begins. Understanding the ebb and flow allows women to embrace their unique biological poetry. The average cycle spans 28 days, with variations such as a 24-day whirl or a 35-day crescendo. The cycle is marked by peaks and troughs, with fertility peaks around mid-cycle, typically Day 14, and potential denouement if fertilization doesn't occur. By embracing this cyclical narrative, individuals can anticipate, understand, and marvel at the intricate choreography of the menstrual cycle.

Managing menstrual hygiene

1. **The Art of Self-Care**: Managing menstrual hygiene is an art—an intimate and powerful discipline that supports both physical and mental well-being. The use of period products, whether pads, tampons, or menstrual cups, becomes a

personal option, providing females with the liberty to decide what corresponds best with their tastes and lifestyle. The art of self-care during menstruation goes beyond product choice—it incorporates habits that promote comfort, hygiene, and general wellness.

2. **Creating a safe atmosphere**: Imagine the atmosphere during menstruation as a sanctuary—a location where girls feel safe, supported, and free from shame. Creating this atmosphere entails open talks about menstruation, debunking misconceptions, and developing a culture that supports the natural cycle of a woman's body. Parents, as nurturers, contribute to this supportive environment by addressing any worries, giving instructions on menstrual hygiene, and reinforcing the concept that menstruation is a natural and normal part of life.

3. **Empowering via knowledge**:
Empowering females via knowledge about menstruation extends beyond biological issues.

It contains conversations about emotional well-being, self-acceptance, and body positivity. By providing girls with information about their bodies and the menstrual process, parents become allies in cultivating a positive mentality and encouraging girls to accept menstruation as a distinct and beautiful element of their femininity.

4. **Celebrating the Feminine Essence**: Menstruation, when seen from the perspective of celebration, becomes a lyrical representation of the feminine soul. It is a moment to recognize the power and resilience inherent in the female body, embracing the cyclical aspect of life. Parents, through supportive interactions and a celebration of menstruation, contribute to the formation of a narrative that reframes this natural occurrence as a source of pride, strength, and connection.

5. **The Beauty of Shared Experiences:** In the chapter on menstruation for girls, envisage a community—a sisterhood where shared

experiences build a tapestry that connects women together. Through open talks, shared knowledge, and an appreciation of the variety of menstrual experiences, girls go on a path of self-discovery that transcends the physical features of menstruation. Parents, as protectors of this story, play a critical role in establishing a feeling of togetherness, understanding, and empowerment.

6. **Embracing the Poetry of Womanhood:** As we dig into the subtleties of menstruation, let's embrace it as the poetry of womanhood—a nuanced and beautiful manifestation of the feminine experience. From comprehending the subtleties of the menstrual cycle to handling period hygiene with grace, this chapter urges girls and their parents to appreciate the natural rhythm of life. May it be a chapter defined by open talks, shared knowledge, and a strong feeling of pride in the unique and transformational experience of menstruation.

7. **Understanding Emotional Changes:** Menstruation isn't only a bodily event; it's a ballet of emotions, a symphony of moods that follows the menstrual cycle. Girls may feel a variety of emotions throughout this period, from heightened sensitivity to reflection. Understanding these emotional shifts becomes a compass, leading females through the many periods of the menstrual cycle with self-compassion and self-awareness.

8. **Embracing Emotional Well-Being**: Parents, as guardians of emotional well-being, play a critical role in developing a happy outlook throughout menstruation. Encouraging open discussion about emotions, giving support during hard periods, and stressing that emotional changes are a natural aspect of the menstrual cycle contribute to the formation of a supportive and understanding atmosphere.

9. **Rituals as Empowerment**: Managing menstrual hygiene goes beyond the practicalities—it incorporates the art of self-care

rituals. Encouraging girls to adopt self-care routines during menstruation, whether it's taking a warm bath, practicing mindfulness, or participating in activities that offer comfort, allows them to connect with their bodies in a positive and supportive manner. These rituals become anchors, anchoring girls in a feeling of self-compassion and resilience.

10. **Educating on Hygiene Practices:** Educating women on good menstrual hygiene habits is a crucial element of this chapter. From the significance of frequent changing of menstrual products to maintaining personal cleanliness, this information lays the basis for a healthy and confident attitude toward menstruation. Parents, as educators, give practical instruction and ensure that girls feel able to handle their menstrual hygiene with confidence.

11. **Debunking Myths and Stigmas:**
In the story of menstruation, dispelling misconceptions and fighting stigmas becomes a

transformational act. Parents help with this process by participating in open talks that debunk myths, normalize the naturalness of menstruation, and build an atmosphere where girls feel comfortable expressing their experiences without guilt or concealment.

12. **Celebrating the Journey**: Celebrate the journey of menstruation as a unique and beautiful manifestation of femininity. Through positive affirmations, shared tales, and a celebration of unique experiences, parents and girls develop a narrative that reframes menstruation as a source of strength, resilience, and connection. This celebration becomes a strong tool for building a happy and empowered mentality around the menstrual cycle.

In the continued investigation of menstruation for girls, let's picture it as a narrative of empowerment—a tale that develops with awareness, self-care, and the celebration of womanhood. This chapter becomes a canvas where parents and girls create an image of strength, perseverance, and self-love. May it be a tale that enables girls to embrace the poetry of their femininity with elegance, confidence, and a strong feeling of pride in the magnificently unique journey of menstruation.

Chapter 6
REPRODUCTIVE SYSTEM EDUCATION

Understanding Reproductive Anatomy

Understanding reproductive anatomy uncovers the miracle of life's blueprint—a sophisticated and intricate design that orchestrates the generation of new life. Reproductive anatomy includes both male and female structures, each performing a distinct part in the path of conception and birth. Picture it as a symphony of organs, hormones, and channels working in unison to continue the beautiful cycle of life.

1. **Female Reproductive Anatomy**: In the world of female reproductive anatomy, consider the uterus as a cradle—a holy area that nourishes and preserves the possibility of life. The fallopian tubes act as delicate bridges, conveying the egg from the ovaries to the uterus. The ovaries themselves are the caretakers of eggs, releasing one each month in a dance that indicates the possibility for fertilization.

2. **Male Reproductive Anatomy**: Male reproductive anatomy develops as a tale of contribution and creation. The testes, like diligent caretakers, create sperm—the tiny builders of life. The sperm's journey is a fascinating one, navigating the complicated pathways of the male reproductive system to meet the awaiting egg, marking the commencement of a new chapter.

The Role of Eggs and Sperm

1. The Dance of Creation:

In the dance of creation, eggs and sperm become the principal players. Eggs, like heavenly spheres, hold the possibility for life inside the ovaries. Their discharge signals the beginning of a delicate trip via the fallopian tubes, where they await the arrival of sperm. Sperm, on the other hand, are the tireless travelers who traverse the male reproductive system with the sole aim of fertilizing the awaiting egg.

2. **Fertilization**:

The Cosmic UnionImagine conception as a celestial union—a combining of genetic material that commences the birth of a unique and amazing person. The meeting of egg and sperm in the fallopian tubes becomes a heavenly dance, signifying the genesis of a new life. This celestial union sets in motion the awe-inspiring process of embryonic development—a voyage that unfolds inside the sanctuary of the uterus.

Empowering Through Education:

Reproductive system education becomes a weapon of empowerment, allowing people the ability to grasp the complicated dynamics of life. Parents, as educators, become mentors in this journey, offering age-appropriate knowledge that demystifies the reproductive system, creating a feeling of wonder, understanding, and respect for the remarkable processes that lead to the production of life.

Fostering open talks: open talks about reproductive anatomy develop a foundation of trust and openness. Parents, by starting talks about the male and female reproductive systems, contribute to the normalcy of this vital component of human development. These interactions create bridges, linking parents and children in a common awareness of the marvels of life.

As we examine reproductive system education, let's spotlight it as a path—an illuminating trip that uncovers the wonders of life's development. Understanding reproductive anatomy, the function of eggs and sperm, and the wondrous processes of creation become essential to understanding the great beauty of life's meticulous design. May this education be a beacon of information, promoting a feeling of wonder, respect, and empowerment in the hearts and minds of people who begin on the illuminating path of reproductive system education.

Chapter 7
PERSONAL HYGIENE AND SELF-CARE

Establishing Good Hygiene Practices

Adolescent well-being is largely influenced by healthy hygiene habits, which encompass physical, emotional, and social aspects. Personal hygiene is a set of daily rituals that promote physical and emotional health, such as frequent washing, dental care, and hair care. Consistency in these routines not only maintains bodily cleanliness but also fosters self-respect and understanding of one's value in overall health. As the body undergoes significant changes, understanding and addressing hygiene needs becomes crucial. Parents, as mentors, play a vital role in raising awareness and encouraging teenagers to adopt hygienic routines as self-care.

Promoting Self-Care During Puberty

1. Holistic Well-Being: Promoting self-care throughout adolescence requires promoting a holistic approach to well-being. Beyond the physical components, it encompasses techniques that help with emotional resilience, stress management, and a healthy self-image. Encourage teens to pursue activities such as mindfulness, writing, and hobbies that bring a feeling of pleasure and satisfaction.

2. Positive Body Image: During puberty, the body experiences changes that may alter an individual's image of themselves. Promoting a good body image becomes an important element of self-care. Parents may help by participating in open talks, highlighting the individuality and beauty of each person, and developing a healthy connection with one's body.

3. **Nurturing Emotional Health:** Self-care extends to emotional health, particularly during the rollercoaster of emotions that commonly follows adolescence. Parents may encourage teenagers to develop coping methods, such as finding social support, participating in creative activities, and practicing self-compassion. These techniques become useful resources for

traversing the emotional environment with resilience.

4. **Recognizing uniqueness**: Cultivating a culture of self-care entails recognizing uniqueness. Each teenager is unique, and their self-care routines may differ. Encourage them to investigate and determine what provides them comfort and pleasure. Whether it's spending time in nature, listening to music, or indulging in creative hobbies, self-care becomes a personal voyage of discovery.

5. **Open conversations:** Establishing open conversations regarding personal hygiene and self-care fosters an atmosphere where teenagers feel comfortable addressing their needs, concerns, and preferences. Parents become partners in this journey, giving direction, listening without judgment, and building a culture that promotes well-being.

Nurturing Well-Being Through Self-Care

This chapter explores personal hygiene and self-care as a journey to cultivate well-being and appreciate uniqueness. It provides guidance on establishing good hygiene habits and creating a culture of self-care that boosts resilience, confidence, and a positive self-image during puberty. The path is defined by self-discovery, self-love, and the development of habits for a lifetime of well-being.

1. Creative Outlets:

Self-care throughout puberty may extend beyond the sphere of personal expression. Encourage teenagers to seek artistic channels that enable them to express themselves. Whether via painting, literature, or other kinds of self-expression, these outlets become therapeutic tools, supporting emotional well-being and offering a healthy conduit for self-discovery.

2. Fashion and Style: The investigation of personal style becomes a way of self-expression. During adolescence, people may find satisfaction in experimenting with clothes and developing their particular sense of style. Parents may assist this discovery by giving direction, accepting individual choices, and establishing an atmosphere where self-expression via dress is appreciated.

3. Physical exercise: Incorporating physical exercise into self-care practices is vital for both physical and emotional well-being. Whether it's indulging in sports, yoga, or other types of exercise, the advantages extend beyond physical health to include stress reduction, increased mood, and greater self-esteem. Parents may support the pursuit of activities that match individual preferences and interests.

4. Healthy Eating Habits: Nutrition plays a significant role in self-care. Encourage good eating habits by offering nutritious meals and snacks. Parents may include teenagers in meal planning and preparation, developing a sensesense of autonomy and responsibility in choosing dietary choices that contribute to overall well-being.

5. Time Management: As teens balance the obligations of school, extracurricular activities, and personal interests, practicing excellent time management becomes a critical element of self-care. Parents may assist in the development of these abilities by giving direction on prioritizing, goal-setting, and building a balanced schedule that allows for both obligations and leisure.

6. **Rest and Relaxation**: Amidst the responsibilities of adolescence, appropriate rest and relaxation are crucial components of self-care. Parents may highlight the significance of excellent sleep, support relaxation methods, and set a bedtime ritual that promotes a peaceful night. Recognizing the benefits of rest as a fundamental pillar of well-being adds to overall physical and mental health.

This chapter explores personal hygiene and self-care as a path to embrace uniqueness, create healthy habits, and balance obligations. It provides a blueprint for teenagers and parents to develop resilience, confidence, and a good sense of self through self-discovery, self-expression, and fostering habits for a lifetime of well-being.

Chapter 8
EMOTIONAL WELL-BEING

<u>Navigating Emotional Changes</u>

Navigating emotional changes throughout puberty is analogous to exploring a wide and varied environment. Adolescents experience a variety of emotions, from pleasure and enthusiasm to doubt and contemplation. Parents play a vital role in building emotional intelligence by encouraging open communication, active listening, and offering direction through the peaks and troughs of emotional exploration.

Communication as a Bridge:

Communication becomes the bridge that unites parents and teenagers across the emotional terrain. Encouraging open talks about thoughts, concerns, and experiences fosters a supportive atmosphere where teenagers feel heard and understood. Parents, as caring guides, navigate these talks with empathy, giving comfort and helping teenagers gain the words to communicate their feelings.

<u>Building resilience and self esteem</u>

Building resilience throughout puberty requires educating teenagers with the skills to manage obstacles and failures. Parents may develop resilience by stressing the value of a growth mindset, fostering problem-solving abilities, and noting that setbacks are chances for learning and progress. This perspective change becomes a cornerstone in establishing resilience—a trait that leads to emotional well-being.

1. **Positive Reinforcement:** Positive reinforcement is a significant technique in cultivating self-esteem. Acknowledging and applauding successes, whether great and little, maintains a good self-image. Parents may help to the building of self-esteem by offering constructive comments, stressing strengths, and establishing an atmosphere that supports a feeling of success and self-worth.

2. **Mindfulness and Emotional Regulation**: Introducing mindfulness techniques becomes a vital component of the emotional well-being journey. Mindfulness helps teenagers gain awareness of their thoughts and feelings, supporting emotional control. Techniques such as deep breathing, meditation, or mindfulness exercises give skills for managing stress, anxiety, and traversing the emotional terrain with a feeling of peace and clarity.

3. **Encouraging Healthy Coping Mechanisms**: Emotional well-being is boosted by appropriate coping skills. Parents may help teenagers in discovering activities that bring consolation and support, whether it's participating in hobbies, spending time in outdoors, or connecting with supportive friends. These processes become key tools in controlling stress and fostering a feeling of balance and emotional harmony.

Emotional well-being is a journey of connection between parents and teenagers, promoting resilience and establishing positive self-esteem. This chapter offers guidance on navigating emotional terrain, celebrating triumphs, and forming habits for a lifetime of emotional well-being, focusing on open communication and habit formation.

Chapter 9
SOCIAL CHANGES AND RELATIONSHIPS

<u>Peer Relationships During Puberty</u>

Peer connections throughout puberty develop as a dynamic tapestry, weaving together threads of shared experiences, growth, and mutual support. Adolescents negotiate the complicated world of friendships, finding new aspects to their social interactions. The essence of these friendships rests not only in company but also in the mutual understanding and camaraderie that grow throughout this transforming time.

As teenagers endure physical, emotional, and social changes, peer connections act as an anchor—a support system where people navigate these changes together. Parents may assist in the formation of strong peer relationships by promoting open communication, teaching empathy, and highlighting the significance of true connections founded on trust and understanding.

Communication with Friends and Family

Open Dialogues: Communication with friends and family becomes a cornerstone of managing social changes throughout adolescence. Encouraging open discussions helps teenagers express their experiences, worries, and successes. Parents, as valued confidants, play a critical role in fostering an atmosphere where teenagers feel comfortable discussing their social relationships, giving assistance, and navigating the subtleties of friendships.

Understanding Family Dynamics: Navigating societal changes goes beyond friendships to incorporate family dynamics. Adolescents and their families endure transformations throughout puberty, and comprehending these changes becomes vital. Open talks about changing responsibilities, expectations, and the necessity of family support help to create a harmonious family dynamic that adjusts to the fluctuating needs of each family member.

Developing Empathy: Developing empathy is a vital component of sustaining good social interactions. Adolescents might benefit from learning the viewpoints and feelings of their classmates and family members. Parents may model empathy through their own interactions, stressing the significance of kindness, active listening, and compassion in developing strong and lasting connections.

Navigating Peer Pressure: Peer pressure is a feature of the social environment throughout puberty. Parents may support teenagers in building resistance to peer pressure by establishing a feeling of self-confidence, imparting critical thinking abilities, and stressing the significance of choosing decisions consistent with their beliefs. Open talks regarding peer pressure provide a setting where teenagers feel empowered to make choices that represent their uniqueness.

Navigating Conflicts: Conflicts are a normal aspect of relationships, and learning to handle them becomes a vital skill. Adolescents benefit from help in resolving disagreements with friends and family members through good communication, empathy, and compromise. Parents, as mediators, may provide skills for dispute resolution and model appropriate communication patterns within the family.

Encouraging Individuality: Nurturing healthy social ties requires valuing uniqueness throughout friendships and family interactions. Adolescents start on a path of self-discovery, and parents may help this by promoting honesty, respecting personal limits, and establishing an atmosphere where each individual feels appreciated for their unique talents.

In the investigation of societal changes and connections, let's see it as a tapestry—a lively and growing fabric woven with strands of friendship, family, and uniqueness. This chapter provides help in navigating the shifting terrain of peer connections and family dynamics throughout puberty. May it be a journey distinguished by open communication, empathy, and the building of connections that lead to a lifetime of happy and meaningful interactions.

Chapter 10

ADDRESSING COMMON CONCERNS AND QUESTIONS

FAQs about Puberty

This section provides answers to common questions (FAQs) teenagers may have about puberty, including physical changes like growth spurts, acne, and voice changes. Parents can provide advice on understanding these changes as natural and offering tips on maintaining hygiene habits. Emotional shifts can lead to mood swings, heightened sensitivity, and emotional management. Addressing these FAQs requires understanding the emotional turmoil, emphasizing open communication, and teaching coping techniques like mindfulness and self-expression. Parents should also remind teenagers that everyone experiences puberty at their own pace and provide support to navigate these changes.

FAQs about puberty

1. FAQ: Why am I having mood swings throughout puberty?

Address: Mood swings are a frequent feature of puberty owing to hormonal changes. It's natural to experience a variety of emotions. Maintaining open communication and finding appropriate outlets for emotions may help manage this element of puberty.

2. FAQ: Is it typical to start puberty sooner or later than my friends?

Address: Yes, it's perfectly typical. Puberty onset varies greatly, and everyone experiences it at their own speed. Emphasize that there's no "right" or "wrong" time for puberty—it's a unique experience for each person.

3. FAQ: Why do I develop acne throughout adolescence, and how can I treat it?

Address: Acne is widespread owing to increased oil production. Encourage a proper skincare regimen, gentle washing, and avoid poking at pimples. Assure them that acne is transitory and can be handled with good hygiene measures.

4. FAQ: Why is my body changing, and is it natural to feel uncomfortable about it?

Address: Your body is changing as part of growing up. Feeling uncomfortable is typical, and it's good to have conflicting feelings. Emphasize that everyone goes through these changes, and it's a normal part of the process.

5. FAQ: Are there techniques to control period pain?

Address: Yes, there are techniques to control period discomfort. Encourage the use of heating pads, mild exercise, and over-the-counter pain medications. It's crucial to discuss freely about periods and give support throughout this time.

6. FAQ: Why am I growing differently than my friends?

Address: Each individual grows at their own speed, and variances in growth are natural. It's crucial to accept and celebrate the uniqueness of your body. Remind them that variability in growth is what makes people distinctive.

Addressing Myths and Misconceptions

This section debunks myths and misconceptions about puberty, focuses on facts, and promotes open discussions between parents and teenagers. It emphasizes the importance of normalizing individual differences and fostering a culture of understanding. Parents should provide comprehensive information beyond physical characteristics, such as relationships, mental health, and self-care. Open communication fosters trust and deepens parent-child bonds, ensuring teenagers feel supported throughout their journey. Addressing issues and queries is a continuous process that requires open interactions. This guide serves as a companion to tackle doubts, dispel falsehoods, and develop a culture of knowledge. It encourages teenagers and parents to navigate the intricacies of puberty with confidence, knowledge, and shared understanding. The chapter aims to help individuals embrace the transforming journey of puberty with curiosity, resilience, and the knowledge that they are not alone in their experiences.

Addressing Puberty Misconceptions

1. Misconception: Puberty occurs overnight.
Address: Puberty is a lengthy process that takes many years. It includes a sequence of physical and emotional changes that emerge over time. Assure teenagers that the changes are natural and happen at their own speed.

2. Misconception: Everyone experiences puberty in the same manner.
Address: Puberty is very individual, and experiences vary. Emphasize that variances in timing, growth, and development are perfectly natural. Celebrate uniqueness and variety.

3. Misconception: You have to conceal your emotions throughout puberty.
Address: It's necessary to communicate feelings honestly. Encourage discussion about emotions, stressing that it's normal to seek help. Dispelling

this misunderstanding helps emotional well-being throughout adolescence.

4. Misconception: Puberty solely includes physical changes.
Address: Puberty covers both physical and emotional changes. It's not only about beauty but also about developing emotional intelligence, creating connections, and navigating a spectrum of emotions.

5. Misconception: Body changes suggest anything is wrong.
Address: Body changes are a normal component of growing up. Assure them that these changes reflect a healthy journey toward maturity. Encourage open conversation to address any issues they may have.

6. Misconception: You should compare your growth to others.
Address: Comparisons might lead to unneeded tension. Remind teens that everyone's path is unique. Emphasize the significance of

self-acceptance and concentrating on their own progress.

These examples demonstrate frequent questions and misunderstandings regarding puberty. Addressing these issues with factual information develops a supportive atmosphere, empowers people, and helps them traverse this transitional era with confidence and knowledge.

Chapter 11
PARENTS' ROLE IN PUBERTY EDUCATION

Open Communication Strategies

Creating a Foundation of Trust:
Parents have a critical role in helping their children through the challenges of puberty. Establishing a foundation of trust is vital. Encourage open communication by establishing a secure atmosphere where teenagers feel comfortable addressing their questions, concerns, and experiences without fear of judgment. Be a supportive listener, validating their sentiments and telling them that their ideas and emotions are genuine.

Initiating talks:
Initiating talks about puberty needs a fine mix of sensitivity and openness. Start talking organically, bringing puberty-related issues into ordinary conversations. Use possibilities like viewing a relevant TV program, reading a book

together, or simply discussing a connected news piece to introduce the topic. This incremental approach eases teenagers into talking about their developing bodies and emotions.

<u>Supporting Your Child Through Puberty</u>
Offering Accurate Information:
Supporting your kid through puberty starts with offering accurate and age-appropriate information. Equip yourself with information about the physical, emotional, and social changes connected with puberty. Be prepared to answer their inquiries with honesty and clarity, using language that is accessible and soothing. Correct any misunderstandings and underline that puberty is a normal part of growing up.

Normalizing the Experience: Normalize the experience of puberty by telling your youngster that everyone goes through it. Share anecdotes of your own experiences or those of family members, underscoring that the path is unique for each person. By normalizing the changes, you help to create a positive mindset and reinforce the concept that puberty is a natural and healthy time of life.

Emphasizing Self-Acceptance: Nurturing a good body image is vital throughout puberty. Encourage self-acceptance by highlighting that bodies exist in many forms and sizes, and these changes are a celebration of uniqueness. Discourage comparisons to artificial standards and foster a positive attitude regarding one's physique.

Celebrating uniqueness: Celebrate your child's uniqueness by appreciating their skills, abilities, and distinctive traits. Reinforce that their value is not primarily defined by physical beauty but by their character, generosity, and the good contributions they make. Fostering a sense of self-worth helps promote a healthy body image and mental well-being.

Encouraging Emotional Expression: Parents have a vital role in establishing emotional intelligence throughout puberty. Encourage your youngster to express their feelings honestly and without judgment. Create an atmosphere where kids feel safe discussing their highs and lows. By noticing and accepting their feelings, you promote emotional resilience and help children navigate the vast world of emotions.

Teaching Coping Methods: Puberty brings significant emotional issues, and teaching coping methods becomes an important element of parental supervision. Introduce practices such as mindfulness, deep breathing, or writing to help your kid handle stress and emotions. By offering methods for emotional regulation, you enable them to negotiate the emotional ups and downs with a feeling of control and self-awareness.

Modeling Respectful Communication: Parents serve as significant role models for good partnerships. Model polite communication in your relationships with your kids and others. Demonstrate active listening, empathy, and constructive conflict resolution. By exhibiting these communication abilities, you create a blueprint for your kid to establish good connections with classmates, family, and, ultimately, in romantic circumstances.

Discussing consent and limits: Puberty is a vital moment to discuss consent and personal limits. Engage in age-appropriate talks about the importance of respecting others' boundaries and the relevance of clear communication in relationships. Equip your youngster with the concept that permission is enthusiastic, ongoing, and may be revoked at any moment.

Navigating Gender and Identity: In the developing landscape of adolescence, debates concerning gender identity and expression may occur. Create an inclusive atmosphere where your kid feels encouraged to develop their individuality. Be open to talks regarding gender diversity, stressing that everyone's path of self-discovery is unique, meaningful, and worthy of respect.

Fostering Acceptance: Foster acceptance and understanding by educating oneself about varied gender identities. If your kid exhibits non-binary or gender-expansive sentiments, approach the subject with kindness and a readiness to learn. Affirm their identity, and if required, seek advice from supporting resources or experts.

This chapter explores the role of parents in puberty education, focusing on a guided journey marked by open communication, support, and self-image development. It serves as a guidebook for parents, offering techniques to manage puberty education issues with empathy and compassion. The aim is to enhance parent-child relationships, encourage good communication, and instill confidence in teenagers as they navigate the changing era of puberty. The chapter emphasizes emotional intelligence, support for healthy relationships, and an inclusive understanding of gender and identity. It provides a compass for parents to navigate the delicate aspects of puberty education with empathy, openness, and dedication to nurturing their child's holistic development.

CONCLUSION

<u>Celebrating Puberty Milestones</u>

As we end our guide to puberty education, it's crucial to appreciate the milestones that characterize this transforming journey. Puberty is a period of enormous growth—physically, emotionally, and socially. Each stage offers distinct difficulties and discoveries, generating a tapestry of experiences that add to the rich mosaic of growing up.

The physical changes that accompany puberty symbolize the extraordinary transformation from infancy to adolescence. Celebrate the growth spurts, the emergence of secondary sexual traits, and the distinctive attributes that make each person remarkable. By celebrating these physical milestones, we confirm the normal growth of the human body and create a feeling of self-acceptance.

Puberty is a period of emotional upheaval and self-discovery. Celebrate the emotional milestones—moments of perseverance, self-expression, and the growth of emotional intelligence. These milestones contribute to the formation of a healthy and flexible emotional foundation, helping people to manage life's complexity with grace and understanding.

The path during puberty entails negotiating connections with friends, family, and oneself. Celebrate the milestones of creating relationships, exhibiting empathy, and recognizing the significance of good communication. By cultivating meaningful connections, people gain the social skills and emotional resilience required to prosper in all facets of life.

Growing up is a unique and personal adventure. Embrace the milestones that showcase individuality—distinct interests, abilities, and opinions. By identifying and honoring individual talents, we build a sense of self-worth that transcends physical appearance, leading to a healthy and resilient sense of identity.

As people negotiate the changing age of adolescence, celebrate the milestones of confidence and self-assurance. Through open communication, correct information, and a supportive atmosphere, people build the resilience to confront difficulties, make educated choices, and handle life's complexity with a feeling of empowerment.

Puberty is simply one chapter in the continuing saga of development and self-discovery. As parents, caregivers, and people, the journey continues with continual support, understanding, and a dedication to continuing learning. Celebrate the milestones of continuing talks, shared experiences, and the ever-deepening relationships that define the maturing relationship between parents and teenagers.

In conclusion, this book serves as a compass for the transforming journey of puberty, recognizing milestones, and embracing the process of growing up. May it be a resource that supports open conversation, deepens understanding, and gives the assistance required to traverse the challenges of adolescence with confidence and resilience. Here's to appreciating the unique journey of puberty and the continuous story of development, self-discovery, and a lifetime of learning.

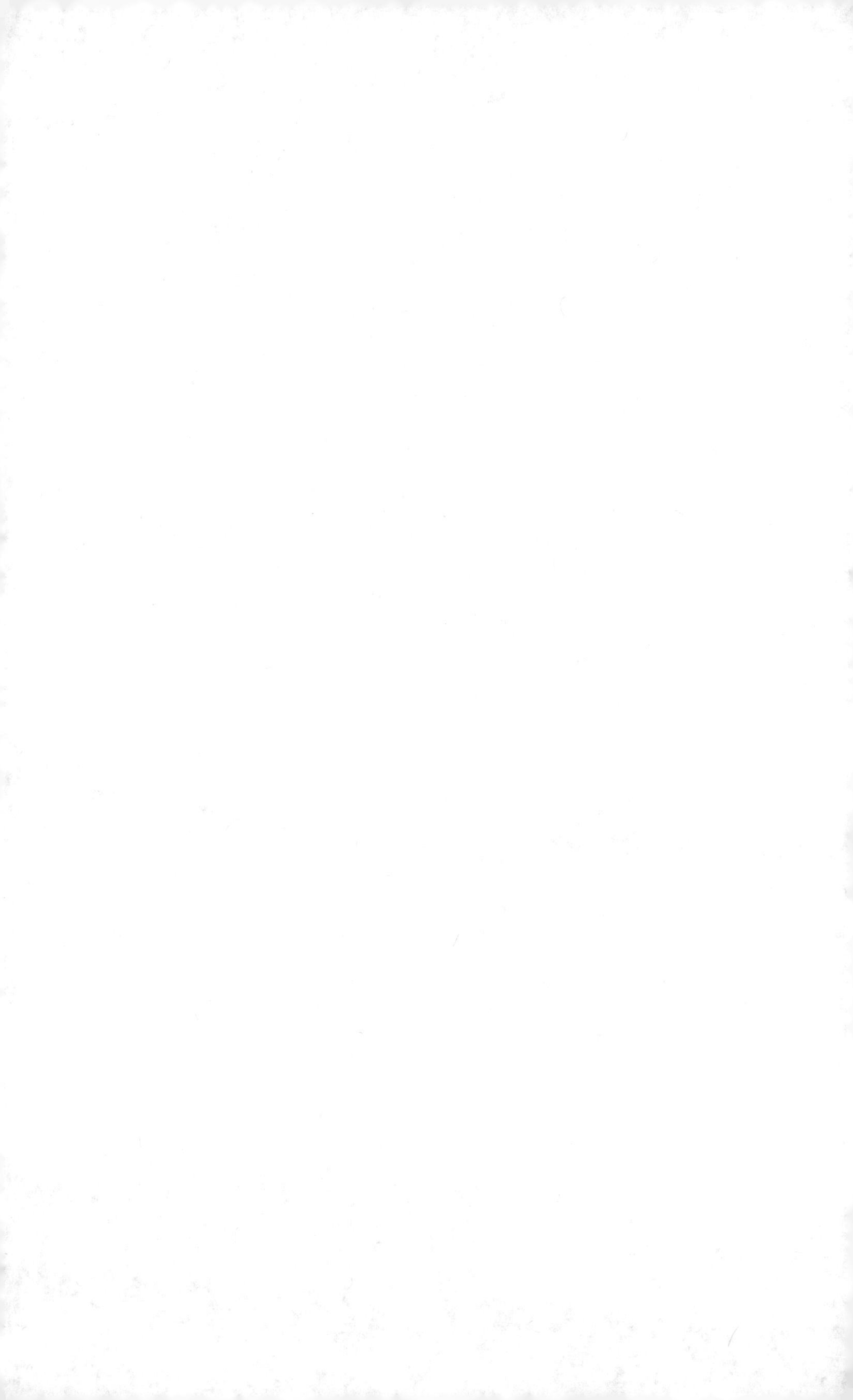

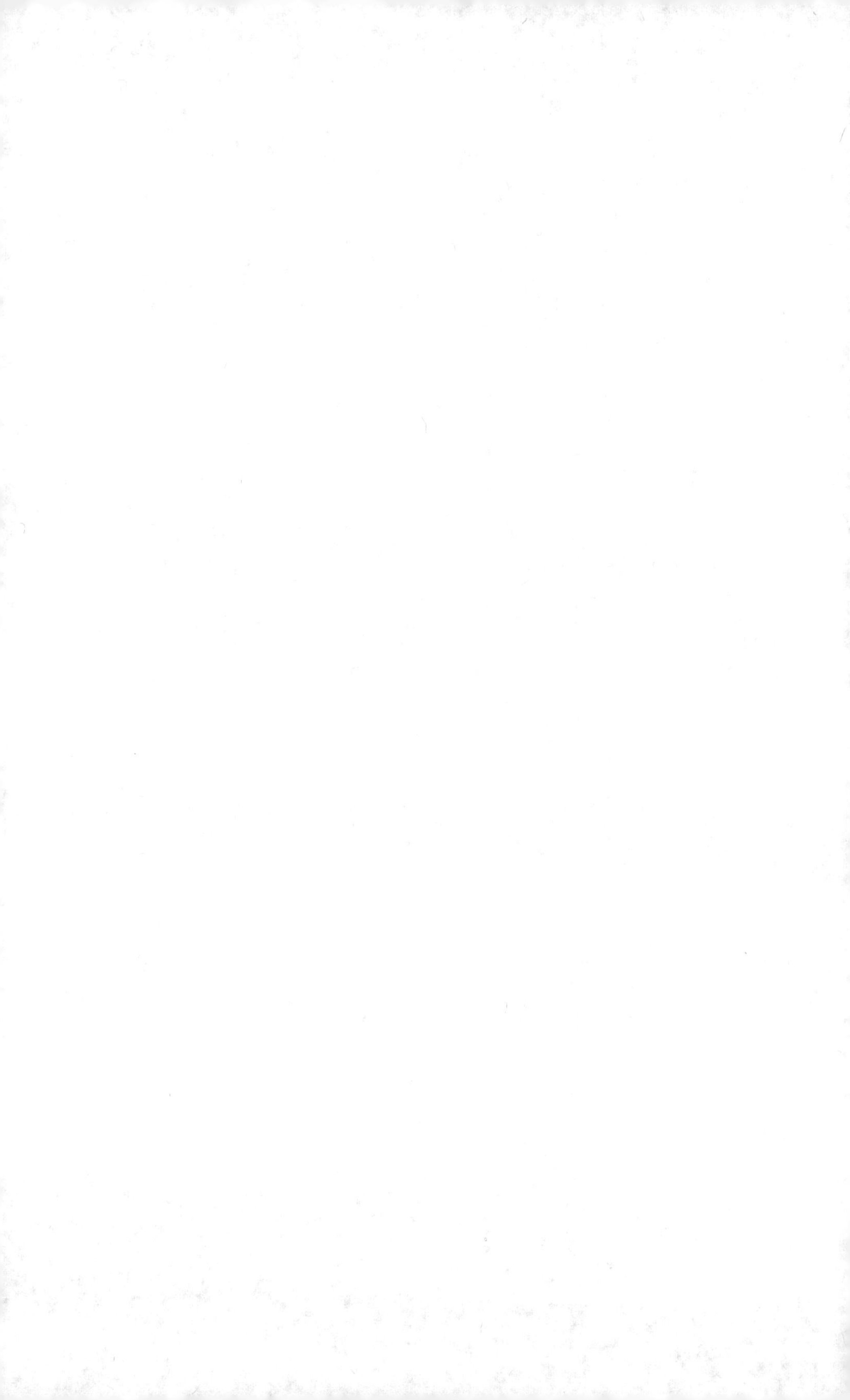